THE COMPLETE ANTI-INFLAMMATORY DIET COOKBOOK FOR BEGINNERS

Soothing Your Body: Easy and Healthy Recipes

MACKI VICKI

TABLE OF CONTENTS

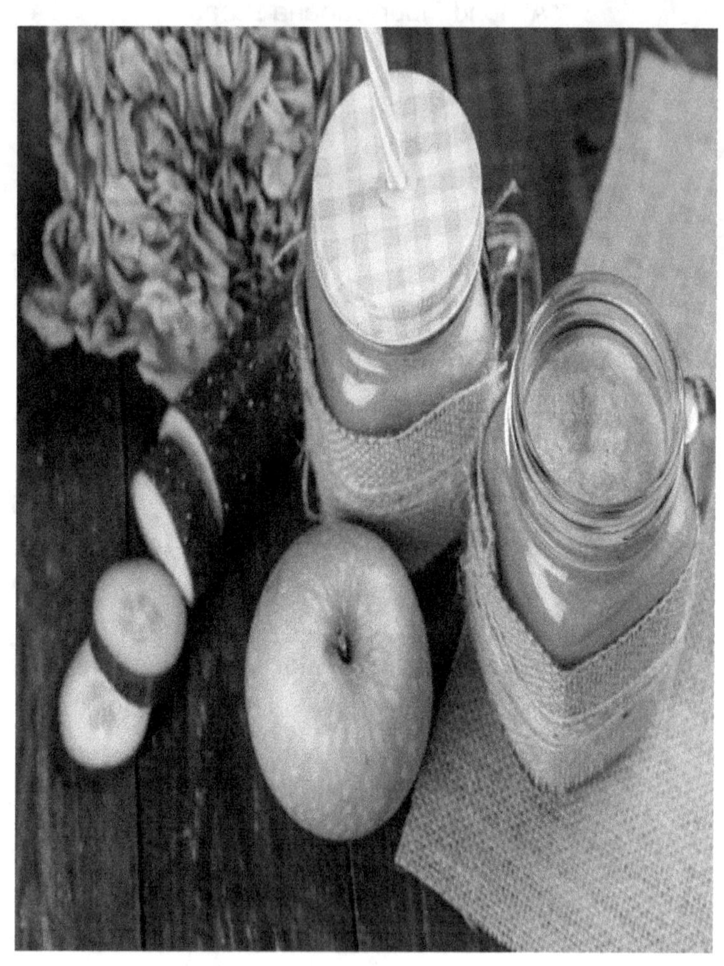

INTRODUCTION

Welcome to "The Complete Anti-Inflammatory Diet Cookbook for Beginners." If you are maintaining this book, you have already taken step one towards a more fit and greater vibrant you. Within these pages, you may embark on a culinary journey that not best tantalizes your taste buds but additionally empowers you to combat inflammation—the silent offender at the back of many chronic fitness troubles.

Inflammation, even though a natural response within the frame, can flip from buddy to foe whilst it will become chronic. It's the underlying factor in conditions consisting of arthritis, coronary heart disorder, diabetes, and even a few cancers. But right here's the good information: what you put on your plate can play a pivotal position in coping with and decreasing irritation.This cookbook is your gateway to discovering the transformative power of an anti-inflammatory eating regimen. It's no longer about deprivation or bland meals; it is about embracing a way of life that nourishes your body and complements your average well-being. Whether you're a pro domestic cook dinner or a kitchen novice, this cookbook is designed with you in mind

What Awaits You:

- **Educational Insights:** Before we dive into the recipes, we're going to provide you with solid information about irritation, how it influences your

health, and why an anti-inflammatory food regimen is critical.
- **Delicious and Nutrient-Packed Recipes:** You'll discover over 100 recipes that aren't only anti-inflammatory however additionally novice-friendly. From hearty breakfasts to savory dinners and tempting desserts, we have been given your everyday food covered.
- **Fresh and Wholesome Ingredients:** Learn a way to choose and put together elements that clearly fight inflammation, such as colorful vegetables, lean proteins, and a host of beneficial herbs and spices.
- **Practical Guidance:** We'll proportion pointers and hints for a successful meal planning, shopping for anti-inflammatory staples, and cooking techniques that maximize health benefits.
- **30-Day Meal Plan:** Kickstart your anti-inflammatory journey with our expertly crafted meal plan. It includes shopping lists and each day menu, taking the guesswork out of your first month.
- **Nutritional Information:** Every recipe comes with precise dietary data, so you can without difficulty music your intake and make informed choices approximately what you consume.
By the time you finish exploring those pages, you may have the knowledge and the tools to make a profound difference on your health. This cookbook is not pretty much converting what's in your plate; it is about changing your life for the higher.
Are you prepared to embrace the scrumptious international of anti-inflammatory cooking? Let's

begin this transformative journey collectively—one meal at a time. Your frame will thank you, and your destiny self will have fun with the choice you are making properly now.

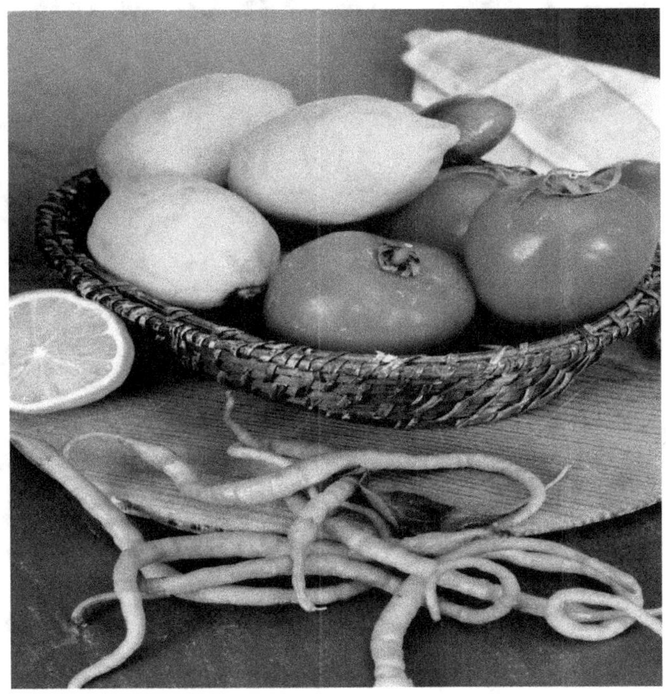

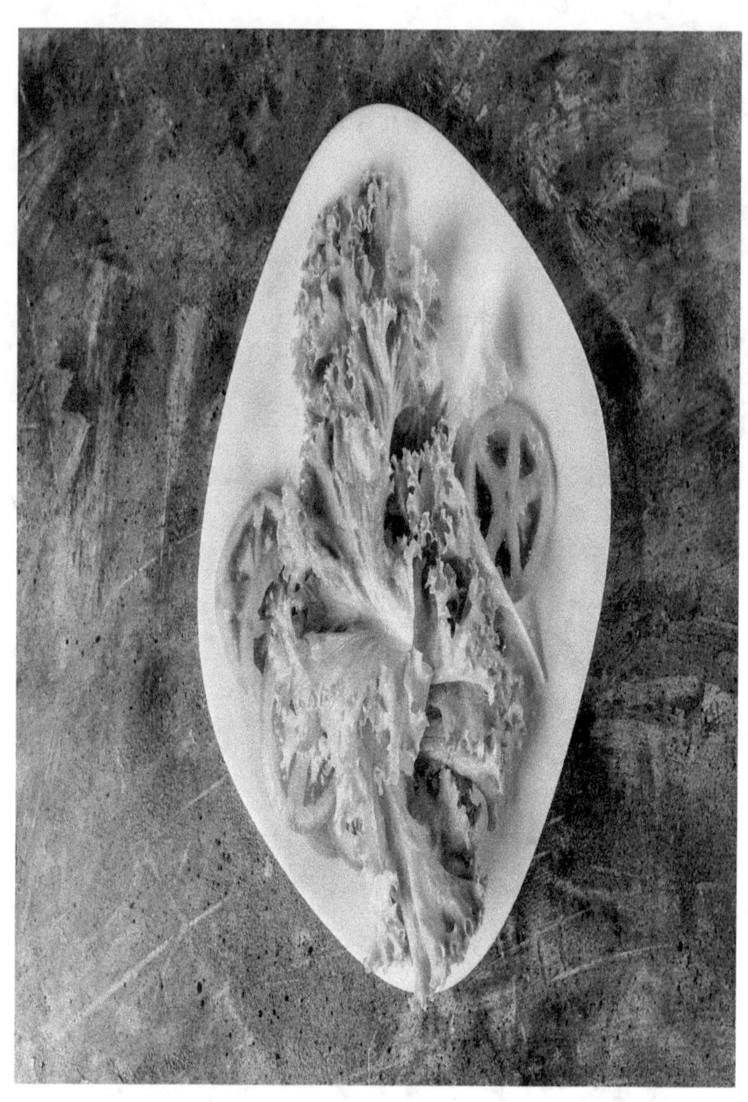

Why Choose an Anti-Inflammatory Diet

International full of dietary tendencies and fads, the anti-inflammatory weight loss program stands proud as a technological knowledge-backed approach to beautify your health and proper-being. Here are compelling reasons why you must not forget embracing an anti inflammatory eating regimen:

One: Reduce Chronic Inflammation:** Chronic irritation is at the basis of many not unusual fitness situations, along with coronary heart disease, arthritis, diabetes, or even cancer. By adopting an anti-inflammatory food regimen, you could successfully lower the levels of infection to your body, potentially decreasing the danger of growing these chronic illnesses.

Two: Alleviate Pain:** If you suffer from situations like arthritis or inflammatory bowel sickness, you apprehend the debilitating ache and pain they could cause. An anti inflammatory weight-reduction plan can assist alleviate a number of these signs by means of lowering infection and enhancing universal joint and gut health.

Three: Boost Your Immune System:** A well-balanced anti-inflammatory weight-reduction plan is wealthy in nutrients, minerals, and antioxidants that reinforce your immune system. This can assist your body to guard towards infections and ailments, retaining you healthier in the end.

Four: Weight Management:** Obesity and excess body fats can trigger persistent inflammation. An anti-inflammatory weight loss plan can support weight loss or protection via selling healthful ingesting conduct and reducing infection-associated weight gain.

Five:Enhance Cardiovascular Health: Chronic irritation is a key contributor to cardiovascular diseases like coronary heart attacks and strokes. Adopting an anti-inflammatory weight loss program can lead to more healthy cholesterol levels, blood stress, and step forward universal coronary heart fitness.

Six: Mental Well-Being:Emerging research suggests a connection among irritation and intellectual fitness problems like despair and tension. By lowering infection through weight-reduction plans, you can enjoy improved mood and mental well-being.

Seven: Increased Energy: Many people record feeling greater lively and much less fatigued when

following an anti-inflammatory weight loss
program. Nutrient-dense foods can provide
sustained electricity for the duration of the day,
decreasing the want for brief fixes like caffeine or
sugary snack

Eight:Digestive Health:An anti-inflammatory food
plan frequently consists of ingredients which might
be gentle on the digestive machine, making it an
exceptional desire for those with gastrointestinal
problems like irritable bowel syndrome (IBS) or acid
reflux.

Nine.Longevity: By decreasing the threat of
persistent sicknesses and promoting overall fitness,
an anti-inflammatory weight-reduction plan may
additionally make a contribution to a longer and
greater fulfilling lifestyles.

Ten:Holistic Well-Being:Beyond the physical
blessings, an anti-inflammatory weight loss
program encourages an aware and holistic
technique to consume. It fosters a deeper
connection among what you devour and the way it
influences your health and vitality.

In summary, choosing an anti-inflammatory food
plan isn't always just about what you eat; it is about
making an investment for your lengthy-time
period,health and well-being. It's a proactive step
toward a healthier, greater vibrant destiny, wherein
you could revel in lifestyles to the fullest.fosters a

deeper connection among what you devour and the way it influences your health and vitality.

Inflammation can affect your health in various ways:

1. Acute Inflammation: Short-term inflammation is a natural response to injury or infection. It help the body heal by increasing blood flow and immune cell activity.

2. Chronic Inflammation: Prolonged inflammation, often due to factors like a poor diet, stress, or autoimmune conditions, can be harmful. It's linked to chronic diseases like heart disease, diabetes, and arthritis.

3. Cardiovascular Health: Chronic inflammation can damage blood vessels and increase the risk of atherosclerosis (hardening of arteries), leading to heart attacks and strokes.

4. Autoimmune Disorders: Inflammation plays a role in autoimmune diseases where the immune system mistakenly attacked healthy tissues, such as in rheumatoid arthritis or lupus.

5. Digestive Health: Conditions like inflammatory bowel disease (IBD) involve chronic gut inflammation, leading to symptoms like abdominal pain and diarrhea.

6. Mental Health: Emerging research suggests a connection between chronic inflammation and mental health disorders like depression and Alzheimer's disease.

7. Obesity: Fat tissue produces inflammatory chemicals, and excess body fat can lead to chronic low-level inflammation, increasing the risk of metabolic disorders.

8. Cancer: Chronic inflammation may contribute to cancer development by promoting DNA damage and cell mutations.

Managing inflammation through a healthy lifestyle, including a balanced diet, regular exercise, stress reduction, and medical treatment when necessary, can help mitigate its adverse effects on your health.

-Getting Started: Tools and Ingredients

Great! Starting an anti-inflammatory diet cookbook for beginners is a healthy and exciting endeavor. Here's a basic list of tools and ingredients to get started.

Tools:

1.Cookware: Invest in quality pots, pans, and baking sheets.

2.Cutlery: Good knives, cutting boards, and kitchen shears are essential.
3.Blender or Food Processor: Useful for making smoothies, sauces, and dips.
4.Measuring Cups and Spoons: Precision in measuring ingredients is key.
5. Grater and Zester: For grating vegetables and citrus.
6.Mixing Bowls: Various sizes for mixing and marinating.
7.Oven and Stovetop: Ensure they are in good working condition.
8.Kitchen Gadgets: Can openers, thermometers, and timers.

Ingredients:

1.Fruits and Vegetables: A wide variety of antioxidants and nutrients.
2.Lean Proteins: Such as poultry, fish, and tofu.
3.Healthy Fats: Avocado, olive oil, nuts, and seeds.
4.Whole Grains: Brown rice, quinoa, oats, and whole wheat.
5.Herbs and Spices: Turmeric, ginger, garlic, and other anti-inflammatory options.
6.Low-Sugar Dairy: Greek yogurt or dairy alternatives.
7.Legumes: Beans, lentils, and chickpeas for plant-based protein.
8.Sweeteners: Honey, maple syrup, or stevia as natural alternatives.

9.Beverages: Green tea, herbal teas, and plenty of water.
10.Condiments: Vinegar, low-sodium soy sauce, and mustard.

Remember to consult with a healthcare professional or nutritionist for personalized advice and recipes tailored to your dietary needs and goals. Enjoy your journey into the world of anti-inflammatory cooking!

-Tips for Success on Your Anti-Inflammatory Journey

Certainly! Success on your anti-inflammatory journey involves more than just the right tools and ingredients.

Here are some important tips:
1.Consult a Healthcare Professional: Before making significant dietary changes, consult with a doctor or nutritionist to ensure it's suitable for your health needs.

2.Educate Yourself: Understand what inflammation is and how it affects your body. Knowledge empowers you to make informed choices.

3.Plan Your Meals: Create a meal plan with a variety of anti-inflammatory foods to ensure you get a balanced diet.

4.Read Labels: Learn to read food labels to identify additives, preservatives, and unhealthy fats that can promote inflammation.

5.Cook at Home: Preparing meals at home gives you control over ingredients and cooking methods.

6.Choose Whole Foods: Opt for whole grains, fresh fruits, and vegetables over processed foods.

7.Healthy Fats: Incorporate sources of healthy fats like avocados, nuts, and fatty fish (e. g. ,salmon).

8. Spice it Up: Use herbs and spices like turmeric, ginger, and garlic, known for their anti-inflammatory properties.

9.Stay Hydrated: Drink plenty of water and consider herbal teas like ginger or chamomile.

10.Exercise Regularly: Physical activity can help reduce inflammation and promote overall health.

11.Manage Stress: High stress levels can trigger inflammation. Practice relaxation techniques like meditation or yoga.

12.Get Adequate Sleep: Aim for 7-9 hours of quality sleep each night to support your body's healing process.

13.Monitor Your Progress: Keep a food diary to track how different foods affect your inflammation levels.

14.Be Patient: It may take time to notice changes in inflammation levels. Consistency is key.

15.Seek Support: Join online communities or support groups for sharing experiences and recipe ideas.

Remember that the anti-inflammatory diet is a long-term commitment to better health. Individual responses may vary, so it's crucial to tailor your approach to your specific needs and seek professional guidance when necessary

1.**Consult a Healthcare Professional**: Before making significant dietary changes, consult with a doctor or nutritionist to ensure it's suitable for your health needs.

2. **Educate Yourself**: Understand what inflammation is and how it affects your body. Knowledge empowers you to make informed choices.

3. **Plan Your Meals**: Create a meal plan with a variety of anti-inflammatory foods to ensure you get a balanced diet.

4. **Read Labels**: Learn to read food labels to identify additives, preservatives, and unhealthy fats that can promote inflammation.

5. **Cook at Home**: Preparing meals at home gives you control over ingredients and cooking methods.

6. **Choose Whole Foods**: Opt for whole grains, fresh fruits, and vegetables over processed foods.

7. **Healthy Fats**: Incorporate sources of healthy fats like avocados, nuts, and fatty fish (e. g. , salmon).

8. **Spice it Up**: Use herbs and spices like turmeric, ginger, and garlic, known for their anti-inflammatory properties.

9. **Stay Hydrated**: Drink plenty of water and consider herbal teas like ginger or chamomile.

10. **Exercise Regularly**: Physical activity can help reduce inflammation and promote overall health.

11. **Manage Stress**: High stress levels can trigger inflammation. Practice relaxation techniques like meditation or yoga.

12. **Get Adequate Sleep**: Aim for 7-9 hours of quality sleep each night to support your body's healing process.

13. **Monitor Your Progress**: Keep a food diary to track how different foods affect your inflammation levels.

14. **Be Patient**: It may take time to see noticeable changes in inflammation levels. Consistency is key.

15. **Seek Support**: Join online communities or support groups for sharing experiences and recipe ideas.

Remember that the anti-inflammatory diet is a long-term commitment to better health. Individual responses may vary, so it's crucial to tailor your approach to your specific needs and seek professional guidance when necessary.

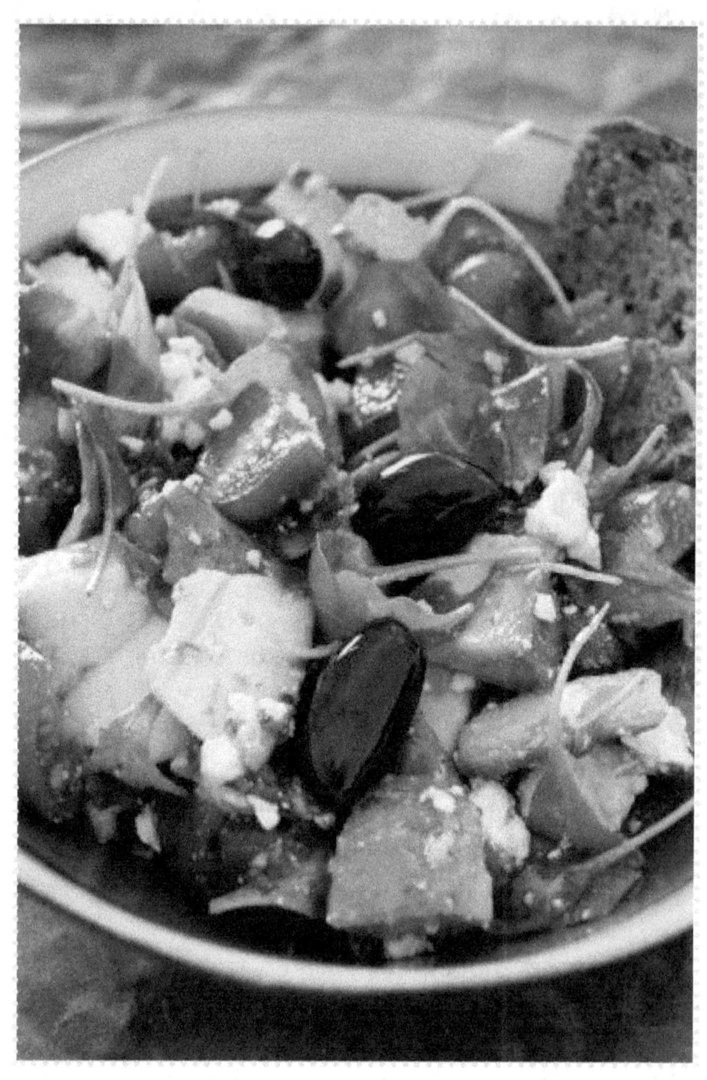

CHAPTER ONE

Breakfast Delights

Begin your day with a burst of anti-inflammatory goodness! This chapter is packed with nutritious and tasty breakfast options that will energize you and set the tone for a day of healthy eating.

Morning Sunshine Smoothie

- Kickstart your morning with this vibrant smoothie packed with antioxidants, vitamin C, and fiber. The perfect way to fuel your day.

Blueberry Almond Overnight Oats

- Prepare your breakfast the night before with these creamy overnight oats. The combination of blueberries and almonds provides a delightful burst of flavor and healthy fats.

Avocado and Egg Breakfast Bowl

- Rich in protein and healthy fats, this savory breakfast bowl is a satisfying way to keep hunger at bay and support your anti-inflammatory goals.

Chia Seed Pudding with Mixed Berries

- Indulge in a guilt-free, sweet treat that's also nutritious. Chia seeds provide Omega-3s and fiber, while mixed berries add natural sweetness and antioxidants.

Each recipe in this chapter is designed to be not only delicious but also easy to prepare, making them ideal for busy mornings. Whether you're a fan of smoothies, oats, savory dishes, or something sweet, you'll find a breakfast delight that suits your taste and helps you on your journey to reducing inflammation. Enjoy a nourishing start to your day!

CHAPTER TWO

** Satisfying Snacks**

Snacking doesn't have to be synonymous with guilt or empty calories. In this chapter, we've curated a collection of satisfying snacks that not only tantalize your taste buds but also support your anti-inflammatory journey. These snacks are perfect for when hunger strikes between meals or when you need an energy boost without the sugar crash. Get ready to discover the joy of healthy snacking.

Roasted Red Pepper Hummus

- Creamy, flavorful, and packed with antioxidants, this homemade hummus is perfect for dipping your favorite veggies or whole-grain crackers.

Greek Yogurt and Cucumber Dip

- A refreshing and protein-packed dip that pairs beautifully with cucumber slices or whole-grain pita chips. It's a cool and satisfying option for warm days.

Spicy Kale Chips

- Crispy, addictive, and surprisingly good for you, these kale chips are seasoned with a hint of spice to satisfy your crunchy snack cravings.

Nut Butter Energy Bites

- Packed with nuts, seeds, and a touch of sweetness, these energy bites are a convenient snack that provides lasting energy and a dose of healthy fats.

Snacking wisely is a key part of maintaining an anti-inflammatory diet. These snack recipes are designed to keep you feeling full and satisfied while nourishing your body with essential nutrients. Say goodbye to mindless munching and hello to snacks that support your health and vitality.

CHAPTER THREE

Vibrant Salads

Salads can be so much more than a bowl of lettuce. In this chapter, we explore the world of vibrant salads that burst with flavor, color, and nutritional goodness. Each salad is carefully crafted to provide a satisfying meal while keeping inflammation at bay. Whether you're a salad aficionado or just starting to embrace leafy greens, these recipes will invigorate your taste buds and your health.

Garden Fresh Greek Salad

- A delightful medley of crisp vegetables, creamy feta cheese, and zesty dressing. This Greek-inspired salad is a true celebration of flavors and textures.

Spinach and Strawberry Salad with Balsamic Vinaigrette

- Sweet strawberries, tender spinach, and a tangy balsamic vinaigrette create a harmonious balance of taste in this refreshing salad.

Quinoa and Roasted Vegetable Salad

- Protein-packed quinoa meets oven-roasted vegetables for a hearty and nutritious salad that's perfect as a standalone meal or a side dish.

Citrus Avocado Salad

- Creamy avocado, juicy citrus segments, and a citrus dressing come together to create a salad that's as beautiful as it is delicious.

Salads are often underestimated, but they can be a satisfying and flavorful part of your anti-inflammatory diet. These recipes prove that salads can be a feast for the senses and a source of vibrant health. Say goodbye to bland greens and embrace the world of exciting, anti-inflammatory salad creations.

CHAPTER FOUR

** Wholesome Soups**

There's nothing quite like a warm bowl of soup to soothe the soul and nourish the body. In this chapter, we dive into the world of wholesome soups that are not only comforting but also brimming with anti-inflammatory ingredients. From rich and hearty broths to velvet vegetable purées, these soups will become your go-to comfort food while supporting your health and wellness.

Tomato Basil Soup

- A classic favorite made even better with the addition of fresh basil. This tomato soup is the perfect blend of comforting and nutritious.

Turmeric and Ginger Carrot Soup

- Vibrant and full of warmth, this carrot soup boasts the anti-inflammatory power of turmeric and ginger, making it a perfect choice for soothing both body and soul.

Chicken and Vegetable Broth

- A homemade broth that's not only the foundation
of many delicious recipes but also a source of
essential nutrients and collagen to support joint
health.

Lentil and Kale Soup

- Loaded with protein, fiber, and leafy greens, this
hearty soup is a satisfying and anti-inflammatory
meal in a bowl.

Warm up from the inside out with these wholesome
soups. Whether you're seeking comfort on a chilly
evening or a nutrient-packed meal to keep you
energized, these recipes will become your trusted
companions throughout your anti-inflammatory
journey.

CHAPTER FIVE

Nourishing Main Courses

Main courses are the heart of any meal, and in this chapter, we present a delightful array of nourishing dishes that take center stage in your anti-inflammatory diet. These recipes are designed to satisfy your taste buds and your health goals simultaneously, proving that eating well can be a delicious adventure.

Baked Salmon with Dill and Lemon

- Succulent salmon infused with the brightness of dill and lemon. This dish is a celebration of flavors and a rich source of omega-3 fatty acids.

Grilled Turmeric Chicken

- Tender, juicy chicken marinated in turmeric and spices, creating a dish that's both vibrant in color and full of anti-inflammatory benefits.

Black Bean and Sweet Potato Tacos

- A plant-based delight that's hearty and satisfying. These tacos are filled with fiber-rich black beans, roasted sweet potatoes, and a medley of colorful veggies.

Quinoa-Stuffed Bell Peppers

- Bell peppers become edible vessels for a quinoa and vegetable medley, offering a burst of flavor and nutritional goodness.

These main course recipes prove that eating an anti-inflammatory diet doesn't mean sacrificing taste or enjoyment. Whether you're a fan of seafood, poultry, or plant-based meals, you'll find nourishing options that will leave you satisfied and feeling fantastic. Get ready to savor every bit of your anti-inflammatory journey.

CHAPTER SIX

Sides and Accompaniments

A well-rounded meal is often defined by its sides and accompaniments. In this chapter, we explore a variety of dishes that complement your main courses and add layers of flavor and nutrition to your anti-inflammatory dining experience. From roasted vegetables to wholesome grains, these sides and accompaniments are the perfect partners for your meals.

Garlic and Herb Roasted Vegetables

- A medley of colorful vegetables roasted to perfection with garlic and aromatic herbs. These veggies are both visually appealing and bursting with flavor.

Cauliflower Rice

- A low-carb alternative to traditional rice, cauliflower rice is a versatile side that pairs wonderfully with a wide range of main courses.

Creamy Mashed Sweet Potatoes

- Creamy, sweet, and rich in vitamins and fiber, these mashed sweet potatoes are a comforting side dish that compliments a variety of proteins.

Sauteed Garlic Spinach

- Quick, simple, and packed with nutrients, this sauteed spinach is a healthy and flavorful way to add greens to your plate.

These sides and accompaniments are more than just supporting acts; they elevate your meals to a whole new level. Whether you're looking for vibrant colors, hearty textures, or subtle flavors, you'll find the perfect addition to your anti-inflammatory feast in this chapter. Prepare to delight in the art of pairing and discover how these dishes can enhance your culinary experience.

CHAPTER SEVEN

** Sweet Treats and Desserts**

A life without indulgence is no life at all, and that's why we've dedicated a chapter to sweet treats and desserts that won't derail your anti-inflammatory efforts. In this section, you'll find guilt-free delights that satisfy your sweet tooth while adhering to your healthy eating goals. These recipes prove that you can have your cake (or in this case, dessert) and eat it too, all while promoting an anti-inflammatory lifestyle.

Berry Chia Seed Parfait

- A colorful and delectable parfait filled with layers of mixed berries, creamy yogurt, and chia seeds for added texture and nutrition.

Dark Chocolate Avocado Mousse

- A velvety, chocolatey delight that combines the richness of dark chocolate with the creamy goodness of avocado. It's a dessert that's as decadent as it is healthy.

Mixed Berry Sorbet

- A refreshing and naturally sweet sorbet made with
a medley of berries. This frozen treat is both
cooling and antioxidant-packed.

Almond Flour Banana Bread

- A moist and nutty banana bread made with
almond flour, offering a gluten-free alternative to
traditional recipes.

Desserts are meant to be enjoyed, and these
recipes ensure you can savor your favorite sweets
without guilt. From creamy parfaits to indulgent
chocolate treats, you'll find desserts that not only
taste fantastic but also align with your
anti-inflammatory journey. Treat yourself while
taking care of your health – it's the best of both
worlds.

CHAPTER EIGHT

** Beverages and Drinks**

Quench your thirst and boost your well-being with the delightful beverages and drinks featured in this chapter. Staying hydrated and enjoying flavorful, anti-inflammatory beverages can be an essential part of your wellness journey. From soothing teas to refreshing smoothies, these recipes will keep you hydrated and satisfied.

Anti-Inflammatory Turmeric Tea

- A warming and comforting tea made with turmeric and spices known for their anti-inflammatory properties. It's the perfect beverage to start or end your day.

Cucumber and Mint Infused Water

- Stay hydrated with this refreshing infused water, featuring the crispness of cucumber and the freshness of mint leaves.

Green Smoothie for Cleansing

- A nutrient-packed smoothie that not only tastes great but also helps detoxify your body and reduce inflammation.

Golden Milk Latte

- A creamy and golden-hud latte made with turmeric, coconut milk, and a touch of honey, providing a comforting and anti-inflammatory drink option.

Beverages play a crucial role in your daily life, and these recipes ensure that your hydration choices align with your anti-inflammatory goals. Whether you're in need of a revitalizing start to your morning or a soothing sip before bedtime, these drinks will keep you both refreshed and health-conscious. Cheers to a hydrated and inflammation-free you!

CHAPTER NINE

** 30-Day Meal Plan**

Embarking on an anti-inflammatory diet is a journey, and were here to guide you every step of the way. In this chapter, you'll find a meticulously crafted 30-day meal plan that takes the guesswork out of meal preparation. We've designed daily menus complete with breakfasts, lunches, dinners, and snacks, along with detailed shopping lists. This meal plan provides structure and variety, ensuring that you stay on track with your anti-inflammatory goals while enjoying a diverse range of delicious foods.

Week 1: Jumpstart Your Journey
- Discover the basics of an anti-inflammatory diet with tasty and easy-to-prepare recipes that set the foundation for your 30-day adventure.

Week 2: Exploring New Flavors
- Expand your palate with a week filled with diverse and flavorful meals that showcase the versatility of anti-inflammatory ingredients.

Week 3: Variety and Balance
- Achieve balance with a mix of protein-rich dishes, plant-based options, and creative combinations that keep you engaged and motivated.

Week 4: Sustaining Your Progress
- Finish strong with nutrient-packed recipes that highlight the long-term benefits of an anti-inflammatory lifestyle.

Each day of this meal plan is thoughtfully crafted to ensure you receive a balanced intake of essential nutrients, fiber, and anti-inflammatory ingredients. By following this plan, you'll not only simplify your meal preparation but also gain a deeper understanding of how to make anti-inflammatory choices on your own. Let this 30-day journey be the start of a lifelong commitment to your health and vitality.

CHAPTER 10

Eating Out and Social Situations**

Section 1: Making Anti-Inflammatory Choices at Restaurants

1.1 **Understanding Menu Options**
 - Decode menus to identify inflammation-friendly choices.
  - Learn to recognize hidden additives or triggers.

1.2 **Communication with Servers**
  - Effective ways to communicate dietary needs to restaurant staff.
  - Tips for requesting modifications to suit the anti-inflammatory diet.
1.3 **Cuisine-Specific Guidance**
  - Strategies for navigating various cuisines (Italian, Asian, etc.).
  - Highlighting anti-inflammatory options in different culinary traditions.

1.4 **Smart Ordering Techniques**
  - Portion control and choosing smaller, nutrient-dense dishes.
  - Balancing protein, healthy fats, and fiber in restaurant meals.

Section 2: Navigating Social Gatherings and Events

2.1 **Preparing for Events**
   - Pre-event strategies for managing expectations and planning.
   - Bringing anti-inflammatory dishes to share with others.
2.2 **Handling Buffets and Potlucks**
   - Making informed choices in buffet settings.
   - Contributing and enjoying potluck-style gatherings.

2.3 **Alcohol and Beverages**
   - Choosing anti-inflammatory drink options.
   - Managing alcohol consumption in social settings.

2.4 **Dealing with Peer Pressure**
   - Techniques for confidently sticking to your dietary choices.
   - Communicating with friends and family about your preferences.

2.5 **Mindful Eating Practices in Social Situations**
   - Staying present and savoring flavors.
   - Avoiding overindulgence in social settings.

2.6 **Socializing Without Food Focus**

- Alternative activities that shift the focus from eating.

- Strategies for fostering connections beyond shared meals.

This chapter provides practical insights and strategies for maintaining an anti-inflammatory diet while eating out or navigating social events. It empowers readers to make informed choices, communicate effectively, and enjoy social situations without compromising their dietary goals.

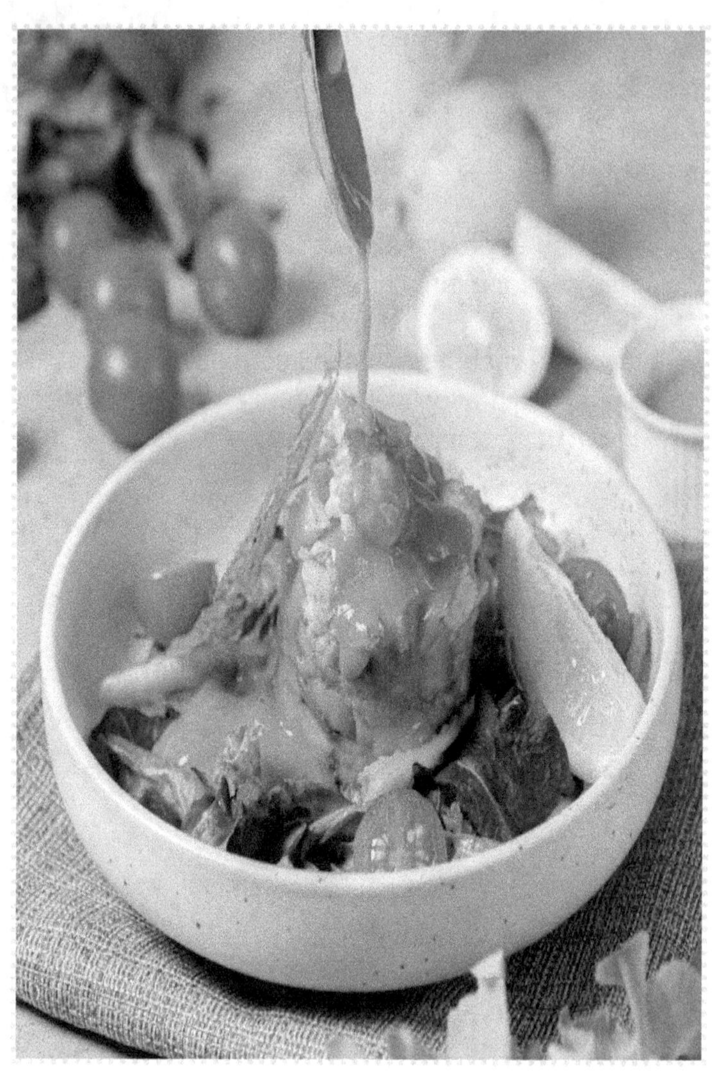

CHAPTER 11

Exercise for Inflammation Reduction**

Section 1: The Role of Exercise in Inflammation Reduction

1.1 **Understanding the Link Between Exercise and Inflammation**
   - Explanation of how regular physical activity influences inflammation.
   - Insights into the positive impact of exercise on overall health.

1.2 **Types of Exercise for Inflammation Reduction**
   - Aerobic exercises: Cardiovascular activities and their anti-inflammatory effects.
   - Resistance training: Building muscle to support the body's inflammatory response.

1.3 **Frequency and Duration Guidelines**
   - Recommendations for the optimal frequency of exercise.

- Balancing intensity and duration for inflammation reduction.

1.4 **Including Flexibility and Mobility Work**
- To improve joint health, perform stretches and mobility exercises.
- Yoga and its role in promoting flexibility and reducing inflammation.

Section 2: Simple Workouts for Beginners

2.1 **Starting with Low-Impact Activities**
- Walking and its underrated benefits for inflammation reduction.
- Cycling and swimming as gentle yet effective exercises.
2.2 **Home-Based Workouts**
- Bodyweight exercises for strength and flexibility.
- Creating a simple yet impactful workout routine at home.

2.3 **Mindful Movement Practices**
- Incorporating mindfulness into exercise for stress reduction.
- Exploring activities like tai chi and qigong for holistic well-being.

2.4 **Building Consistency and Gradual Progress**
- Setting realistic fitness goals for beginners.

- The importance of gradual progression to avoid burnout and injuries.

2.5 **Adapting Exercise to Individual Fitness Levels**
   - Tailoring workouts for different fitness levels and abilities.
   - Modifying exercises based on specific health considerations.

Section 3: Integrating Exercise into Daily Life

3.1 **Incorporating Physical Activity Throughout the Day**
   - Strategies for staying active in sedentary environments.
   - Micro-exercises and movement breaks for desk-bound individuals.

3.2 **Social and Community Exercise**
   - Joining group activities and classes for motivation.
   - The positive impact of social connections on exercise adherence.

3.3 **Creating a Sustainable Exercise Routine**
   - Designing a well-rounded fitness plan for long-term success.
   - Balancing different types of exercise for comprehensive health benefits.

This chapter provides a detailed exploration of the relationship between exercise and inflammation reduction, offering practical advice for individuals at various fitness levels. It guides beginners through simple yet effective workouts, emphasizes the importance of consistency, and encourages the integration of physical activity into daily life for long-term health benefits.

CONCLUSION

Congratulations on completing your journey through "The Complete Anti-Inflammatory Diet Cookbook for Beginners. " You've embarked on a path to better health, and we hope this cookbook has empowered you to make delicious, nutritious choices that support your well-being.

As you conclude this culinary adventure, here are some key takeaways to carry forward:

1. Mindful Eating: Embrace the practice of mindful eating. Pay attention to how your body responds to different foods, savor each bite, and listen to your hunger and fullness cues.

2. Variety is Key: The world of anti-inflammatory eating is diverse and exciting. Continue to explore new ingredients, flavors, and recipes to keep your meals interesting and enjoyable.

3. Sustainable Choices: An anti-inflammatory diet isn't a temporary fix; it's a lifestyle. Make sustainable choices that you can maintain in the long run.

4. Balance and Moderation: While reducing inflammation is essential, remember that balance and moderation are crucial. Occasional treats and deviations from the plan are okay as long as they don't become the norm.

5. Empowerment: You now possess the knowledge and skills to make informed dietary choices that benefit your health. Use this empowerment to advocate for your well-being.

6. Community and Support: Consider joining a community of like-minded individuals who share your dietary goals. Support and encouragement from others can be invaluable on your journey.

Remember that your health is a lifelong journey,and what you eat plays a pivotal role in that journey. Continue to prioritize whole, nutrient-rich foods,stay curious about new culinary experiences,and celebrate the small victories along the way.
We hope this cookbook has not only provided you with delicious recipes but also inspired you to make positive changes in your life. Your body and future self will thank you for investing in your health and well-being. Here's to a vibrant, inflammation-free future!

"Thank you for embarking on this journey toward a healthier, inflammation-free life with 'The Complete Anti-Inflammatory Diet Cookbook for Beginners.' Your commitment to well-being is inspiring. As you explore these pages filled with nourishing recipes, practical tips, and empowering insights, remember that each choice brings you closer to a vibrant, healthier you. Here's to savoring good health, one delicious and anti-inflammatory meal at a time. Thank you for making this cookbook a part of your wellness story!"

www.ingramcontent.com/pod-product-compliance
Lightning Source LLC
Chambersburg PA
CBHW071003260726
48661CB00007B/2762